Eat Well, Live Well: Unleashing the Power of Nutritious Foods for a Vibrant Life

Table of contents

Chapter 1. Understanding Macronutrients and micronutrients 2

Chapter 2: The Role of Fiber: Promoting Digestive Health and Weight Management...2
Chapter 3: Hydration and its Importance for Overall Health 2
Chapter 4: The Power of Antioxidants: Protecting Against Free Radicals and Chronic Diseases..2
Chapter 5: Super Foods: Nutrient-Rich Foods for Optimal Health....2
Chapter 6. Cooking and Food Preparation Techniques for Nutrient Retention...2
Chapter 7: Understanding Food Labels and Making Informed Choices 2
Conclusion: 2
Introduction 1

Introduction:

In today's fast-paced world, where convenience foods and sedentary lifestyles have become the norm, the importance of nutrition cannot be overstated. What we eat directly influences our health and well-being, playing a crucial role in our physical, mental, and even emotional state.
The impact of nutrition reaches far beyond mere sustenance. Our bodies require a complex blend of macronutrients, micronutrients, and other essential components to function optimally. When we provide our bodies with the right balance of nutrients, we unlock a powerful tool for promoting overall health, preventing diseases, and experiencing vibrant living.
The connection between nutrition and health has been recognized since ancient times. The famous quote by Hippocrates, "Let food be thy medicine and medicine be thy food," highlights the profound influence of our dietary choices on our well-being. Scientific research has further substantiated this ancient wisdom, revealing the intricate

ways in which nutrition impacts every aspect of our lives.

Proper nutrition is the cornerstone of a healthy lifestyle. It fuels our bodies, providing the energy and nutrients necessary for daily activities, growth, and repair. It strengthens our immune system, enabling us to ward off illnesses and infections. It supports optimal brain function, enhancing cognitive abilities, focus, and mental clarity. It contributes to healthy weight management, reducing the risk of obesity and related conditions. It promotes cardiovascular health, lowers the chances of chronic diseases such as diabetes, hypertension, and heart disease. It even influences our mood, contributing to emotional well-being and a positive outlook on life.

However, in today's information-saturated world, navigating the vast landscape of nutrition can be overwhelming. Fad diets, conflicting advice, and misinformation abound, making it challenging to distinguish between genuine nutritional principles and mere trends. That is why this comprehensive guide has been created to provide you with a reliable roadmap to healthy eating and vibrant living.

Throughout the chapters of this book, we will explore the fundamental components of nutrition, unravel the mysteries of macronutrients and micronutrients, delve into the benefits of superfoods, and unveil the secrets of mindful eating. We will discuss the importance of hydration, the impact of antioxidants, and the role of fiber in promoting digestive health. You will discover practical tips for meal planning, cooking techniques that maximize nutrient retention, and strategies for making informed food choices.

Whether you are seeking to improve your overall health, manage your weight, boost your energy levels, or simply adopt a more nourishing approach to life, this guide will empower you with the knowledge and tools needed to unleash the power of nutritious foods.

Are you ready to embark on a transformative journey that will revolutionize your relationship with food and revitalize your well-being? Let's dive in and discover how eating well can truly allow us to live well.

Chapter 1. Understanding Macronutrients and micronutrients

A. Macronutrients
1. Carbohydrates:

Carbohydrates are one of the primary sources of energy for our bodies. They can be categorized into two main types: simple carbohydrates and complex carbohydrates. Simple carbohydrates, often referred to as simple sugars, are found in foods like fruits, honey, and processed sweets. They are quickly digested and can cause a rapid spike in blood sugar levels. On the other hand, complex carbohydrates are made up of long chains of sugar molecules and are found in foods such as whole grains, legumes, and vegetables. These carbohydrates are digested more slowly, providing a steady release of energy and helping to maintain stable blood sugar levels.

When it comes to carbohydrates, it's important to focus on consuming complex carbohydrates, as they are typically higher in fiber, vitamins, and minerals compared to simple carbohydrates. Fiber, a type of carbohydrate that cannot be digested by the body, plays a crucial role in promoting healthy digestion, managing weight, and reducing the risk of chronic diseases like heart disease and type 2 diabetes. Incorporating a variety of whole grains, fruits, vegetables, and legumes into our diet ensures we obtain an adequate amount of beneficial carbohydrates and fiber.

2. Proteins:

Proteins are essential for the growth, repair, and maintenance of body tissues. They are composed of smaller units called amino acids, which our bodies need to build and maintain muscles, organs, enzymes, and hormones. Proteins are found in both animal-based and plant-based sources. Animal sources of protein include meat, poultry, fish, eggs, and dairy products, while plant-based sources include legumes, tofu, tempeh, nuts, and seeds.

It's important to consume a variety of protein sources to ensure an adequate intake of all the essential amino acids our bodies require. Some protein sources, such as meat and dairy products, are considered complete proteins as they contain all the essential amino acids in the right proportions. Plant-based protein sources, except soy and quinoa, are generally considered incomplete proteins. However, by combining different plant-based protein sources throughout the day, such as legumes and grains, we can obtain all the necessary amino acids and achieve a complete protein profile.

3. Fats:

Fats often have a negative reputation, but they are an essential macronutrient that our bodies rely on for various functions. Fats provide a concentrated source of energy, help absorb fat-soluble vitamins (A, D, E, and K), support brain function, protect organs, and contribute to hormone production. It's important to understand the different types of fats and make wise choices.

Saturated fats, primarily found in animal products like meat and dairy, as well as some tropical oils like coconut oil, are generally considered less healthy when consumed in excess. They have been associated with an increased risk of heart disease. On the other hand, unsaturated fats, including monounsaturated and polyunsaturated fats, are considered heart-healthy. They are found in foods like avocados, nuts, seeds, olive oil, and fatty fish. Omega-3 and omega-6 fatty acids, which are polyunsaturated fats, play crucial roles in brain health, reducing inflammation, and supporting heart health.

Trans fats, typically found in processed and fried foods, should be avoided as much as possible. They are known to raise LDL (bad) cholesterol levels and increase the risk of heart disease.

4. Balancing Macronutrients:
Balancing macronutrients is essential to support our individual health goals and overall well-being. The optimal macronutrient ratio varies based on factors such as age, sex, activity level, and specific health needs. Generally, a well-balanced diet includes a moderate intake of carbohydrates, a sufficient amount of protein, and healthy fats, tailored to individual needs.

For example, individuals engaged in intense physical activity or athletes may require a higher proportion of carbohydrates to fuel their performance and replenish glycogen stores. On the other hand, those focusing on weight management or following a low-carb approach may opt for a higher proportion of healthy fats and moderate protein intake.

Finding the right macronutrient balance often involves experimentation and listening to our bodies. It can be helpful to consult with a registered dietitian or nutritionist who can provide personalized guidance based on specific goals and health conditions. Additionally, tracking macronutrient intake using food diary apps or journals can provide insights into our dietary patterns and help us make adjustments as needed.

5. **Practical Tips for Incorporating Macronutrients:**

Incorporating macronutrients into our daily meals can be both enjoyable and nutritious. Here are some practical tips to help achieve a balanced macronutrient intake:

- **Focus on whole, minimally processed foods:** Whole grains, lean proteins, and healthy fats should form the foundation of your meals. Choose foods that are as close to their natural state as possible, as they tend to be higher in nutrients and fiber.
- **Prioritize fiber-rich carbohydrates:** Opt for complex carbohydrates such as whole grains, fruits, and vegetables, which provide a steady release of energy and are rich in fiber. Fiber not only aids digestion but also promotes satiety and helps regulate blood sugar levels.
- **Include a source of protein with each meal:** Incorporate lean proteins like poultry, fish, legumes, tofu, or plant-based protein sources in each meal. Protein helps maintain muscle mass, supports cell repair, and keeps you feeling full and satisfied.
- **Choose healthy fats:** Include sources of healthy fats like avocados, nuts, seeds, olive oil, and fatty fish in your diet. These fats provide essential fatty acids and promote satiety. Remember to moderate your

fat intake, as fats are higher in calories compared to carbohydrates and proteins.

- **Practice portion control:** Pay attention to portion sizes to ensure you're getting an appropriate balance of macronutrients. Use measuring cups, scales, or visual cues (e.g., palm-sized portions for protein) to gauge appropriate amounts.
- **Experiment with different meal combinations:** Incorporate a variety of ingredients and flavors to make meals exciting and satisfying. Aim for a colorful plate filled with a mix of macronutrients, including plenty of vegetables, to ensure a nutrient-rich meal.
- **Stay hydrated:** While not a macronutrient, proper hydration is essential for overall health. Water supports digestion, nutrient absorption, and cellular function. Aim to drink adequate water throughout the day and consider hydrating foods like fruits and vegetables.

Understanding macronutrients and their roles in our bodies is fundamental to achieving a balanced and nourishing diet. By incorporating the right balance of carbohydrates, proteins, and fats, we can provide our bodies with the energy and nutrients needed to thrive. Remember, individual needs may vary, and it's essential to listen to your body and make adjustments accordingly. By implementing practical tips and focusing on whole, nutrient-dense foods, we can optimize our macronutrient intake and pave the way for healthy eating and vibrant living.

B. Micronutrients: The Essential Vitamins and Minerals

While macronutrients play a crucial role in providing energy and supporting basic bodily functions, they cannot work effectively without the assistance of micronutrients. Micronutrients include vitamins and minerals, which are required in smaller quantities but are essential for optimal health and well-being.

1. Vitamins:

Vitamins are organic compounds that are necessary for various biological processes in our bodies. They act as coenzymes or cofactors, assisting in numerous chemical reactions that contribute to growth, development, and overall health. There are two main types of vitamins: water-soluble vitamins (such as vitamins C and B vitamins) and fat-soluble vitamins (including vitamins A, D, E, and K). Water-soluble vitamins are not stored in the body for long periods and need to be replenished regularly through our diet. They play essential roles in energy metabolism, immune function, and maintaining the health of our skin, eyes, and nervous system. Good food sources of water-soluble vitamins include fruits, vegetables, whole grains, legumes, and lean proteins. Fat-soluble vitamins, on the other hand, are stored in our body's fat tissues and can be utilized over an extended period. They require dietary fats for absorption and are essential for functions such as vision, bone health, blood clotting, and antioxidant protection. Food sources of fat-soluble vitamins include fatty fish, dairy products, eggs, and certain plant oils.

2. Minerals:

Minerals are inorganic elements that are vital for various bodily functions, including building strong bones and teeth, maintaining fluid balance, transmitting nerve signals, and supporting enzyme activities. There are two main categories of minerals: macrominerals and trace minerals. Macrominerals, required in larger quantities, include calcium, phosphorus, magnesium, sodium, potassium, and chloride. These minerals are essential for bone health, fluid balance, muscle function, and nerve transmission. Food sources rich in macrominerals include dairy products, leafy greens, nuts, seeds, whole grains, and legumes.

Trace minerals, needed in smaller amounts, include iron, zinc, copper, selenium, iodine, manganese, and others. Despite their smaller quantities, these minerals are crucial for enzyme function, hormone synthesis, immune function, and antioxidant defense. Food sources of trace minerals include seafood, nuts, seeds, whole grains, and certain fruits and vegetables.

3. Meeting Micronutrient Requirements:

To ensure we meet our micronutrient requirements, it is important to consume a varied and balanced diet. Incorporating a wide range of fruits, vegetables, whole grains, lean proteins, and healthy fats can help provide a diverse array of vitamins and minerals. However, certain micronutrients may require special attention.

For example, vitamin D is primarily synthesized in the body through exposure to sunlight, but it can also be obtained from fortified foods and fatty fish. Iron, an essential mineral for oxygen transport, is found in both animal-based sources (such as red meat and poultry) and plant-based sources (like legumes, tofu, and fortified grains). Vegetarians and vegans should pay attention to adequate intake and consider sources of vitamin B12, which is predominantly found in animal products.

Understanding cooking methods, food preparation, and storage practices can also help preserve the micronutrient content in our food. Certain vitamins, such as vitamin C, are sensitive to heat and can be lost during cooking. On the other hand, some minerals, like calcium, may be better absorbed when consumed alongside vitamin D or foods high in vitamin C, such as citrus fruits or leafy greens.

In cases where it is challenging to meet micronutrient needs through diet alone, dietary supplements can be considered. However, it is important to consult with a healthcare professional or registered dietitian before starting any supplementation regimen to ensure individual needs are met without exceeding safe levels.

4. Micronutrients and Health:
Micronutrients play a vital role in maintaining overall health and preventing nutrient deficiencies. Deficiencies in certain vitamins and minerals can lead to various health problems. For example, inadequate intake of vitamin C can result in scurvy, while insufficient iron intake can lead to iron-deficiency anemia. Additionally, deficiencies in vitamin D and calcium can contribute to weak bones and an increased risk of osteoporosis.
On the other hand, consuming an adequate amount of micronutrients can have numerous health benefits. For instance, vitamin A supports healthy vision, vitamin C boosts immune function, vitamin E acts as an antioxidant, and vitamin K contributes to blood clotting. Minerals like calcium and phosphorus are crucial for bone health, while potassium helps maintain healthy blood pressure levels.

5. Balancing Micronutrient Intake:
While it is important to ensure adequate intake of essential vitamins and minerals, it is also crucial to avoid excessive intake, as some micronutrients can be toxic in high amounts. This is particularly true for fat-soluble vitamins, as they can accumulate in the body over time.
To achieve a balanced micronutrient intake, focus on consuming a variety of nutrient-dense foods from different food groups. Aiming for a "rainbow" of fruits and vegetables can help ensure a wide range of vitamins and minerals. Additionally, incorporating sources of lean proteins, whole grains, dairy or

dairy alternatives, and healthy fats can further enhance micronutrient intake. Micronutrients, including vitamins and minerals, are essential for supporting overall health and well-being. They play critical roles in numerous bodily functions and are necessary for the growth, development, and optimal functioning of various systems within our bodies. By consuming a varied and balanced diet that includes a wide range of nutrient-dense foods, we can ensure adequate intake of these micronutrients. Whether through fruits and vegetables, whole grains, lean proteins, or healthy fats, every bite we take contributes to unlocking the power of micro nutrition and promoting vibrant living.

Chapter 2: The Role of Fiber: Promoting Digestive Health and Weight Management

Fiber, often referred to as roughage or bulk, is a type of carbohydrate that our bodies cannot fully digest or absorb. Despite this, it plays a crucial role in promoting digestive health, supporting weight management, and contributing to overall well-being.

A. Understanding Fiber:
Fiber is classified into two main types: soluble fiber and insoluble fiber. Soluble fiber dissolves in water and forms a gel-like substance in the digestive tract. It can be found in foods like oats, barley, legumes, fruits, and

vegetables. Insoluble fiber, on the other hand, does not dissolve in water and adds bulk to the stool, aiding in regular bowel movements. It is commonly found in whole grains, nuts, seeds, and the skins of fruits and vegetables.

Both types of fiber have unique properties and contribute to various aspects of digestive health. Soluble fiber helps slow down digestion, promoting a feeling of fullness and reducing appetite. It also helps to stabilize blood sugar levels, as it slows down the absorption of glucose. Insoluble fiber, with its bulk-forming ability, helps prevent constipation by adding bulk to the stool and facilitating regular bowel movements.

B. Benefits of Fiber:

1. Digestive Health:

Fiber plays a vital role in maintaining a healthy digestive system. It helps prevent constipation by softening the stool and promoting regular bowel movements. Additionally, fiber can help prevent or alleviate conditions such as diverticulosis and hemorrhoids by keeping the digestive tract functioning optimally. By promoting healthy gut bacteria, fiber also contributes to a balanced and thriving gut microbiome, which is essential for overall health and immune function.

2. Weight Management:

Including an adequate amount of fiber in our diet can be beneficial for weight management. High-fiber foods tend to be more filling, leading to a decreased overall calorie intake. Fiber-rich meals can promote satiety and reduce the likelihood of overeating or snacking on unhealthy foods. Additionally, the slower digestion of fiber-rich foods can help stabilize blood sugar levels, preventing sharp spikes and crashes that may lead to increased cravings.

3. Heart Health:

A fiber-rich diet has been associated with a reduced risk of heart disease. Soluble fiber, in particular, can help lower LDL (bad) cholesterol levels by binding to cholesterol in the digestive tract and preventing its absorption. By reducing LDL cholesterol, fiber contributes to the maintenance of healthy blood vessels and may help lower the risk of cardiovascular events.

4. Blood Sugar Control:

Fiber plays a significant role in managing blood sugar levels, especially for individuals with diabetes. Soluble fiber slows down the absorption of glucose, preventing rapid spikes in blood sugar levels after meals. This can contribute to better glycemic control and help individuals with diabetes maintain stable blood sugar levels.

C. Incorporating Fiber into Your Diet:

To reap the benefits of fiber, it is important to include a variety of fiber-rich foods in our daily diet. Here are some practical ways to incorporate fiber into your meals:

1. Choose Whole Grains:

Opt for whole grain options such as whole wheat, brown rice, quinoa, and oats. These grains retain their bran and germ layers, which are rich in fiber. Replace refined grains with whole grain alternatives in your meals and snacks.

2. Include Fruits and Vegetables:
Fruits and vegetables are excellent sources of fiber. Aim to include a variety of colorful fruits and vegetables in your diet. Leave the skin on when possible, as it contains a significant amount of fiber. Be creative and add fruits and vegetables to your meals, salads, smoothies, or snacks.

3. Embrace Legumes:
Legumes, including beans, lentils, and chickpeas, are fantastic sources of both soluble and insoluble fiber. Add them to soups, stews, and salads, or use them as a base for plant-based dishes.

4. Snack on Nuts and Seeds:
Nuts and seeds, such as almonds, chia seeds, flaxseeds, and sunflower seeds, are not only rich in healthy fats but also provide a good amount of fiber. Enjoy them as a snack or sprinkle them over salads, yogurt, or oatmeal.

5. Be Mindful of Processed Foods:
Processed foods often lack fiber due to the refining process. Limit your intake of processed snacks, sugary cereals, and white bread, and instead, opt for whole food alternatives that are higher in fiber.

6. Increase Fiber Intake Gradually:
If you are not accustomed to a high-fiber diet, it's important to increase your fiber intake gradually. Sudden and significant increases in fiber consumption can lead to digestive discomfort. Gradually introduce fiber-rich foods and drink plenty of water to help your body adjust.

D. Additional Tips for Fiber Consumption:

Here are some additional tips to make the most of your fiber intake:

- **Stay Hydrated:** Fiber absorbs water, so it's important to drink enough fluids throughout the day to prevent constipation and promote optimal digestion.
- **Read Food Labels:** When grocery shopping, read food labels to identify products that are high in fiber. Look for foods with a higher fiber content per serving.
- **Cook with Herbs and Spices:** Enhance the flavor of your meals by using herbs and spices instead of relying solely on added fats or sauces. This can help reduce calorie intake while still enjoying tasty and fiber-rich dishes.
- **Practice Portion Control:** While fiber is beneficial, it's important to practice portion control to maintain a balanced diet. Pay attention to portion sizes and aim for a well-rounded plate that includes a mix of macronutrients.

Fiber is an essential component of a healthy diet, providing numerous benefits for digestive health, weight management, heart health, and blood sugar control. By incorporating fiber-rich foods such as whole grains, fruits, vegetables, legumes, nuts, and seeds, we can enjoy the advantages of fiber while promoting overall well-being. Remember to increase fiber intake gradually, stay hydrated, and make mindful food choices to optimize your fiber consumption. With the power of fiber on your side, you can support a healthy digestive system and maintain a balanced approach to weight management.

Chapter 3: Hydration and its Importance for Overall Health

Water is an essential component of our bodies, comprising a significant percentage of our overall weight. Adequate hydration is crucial for maintaining optimal bodily functions, supporting various physiological processes, and promoting overall health.

A. The Role of Water in the Body: Water plays a vital role in maintaining and regulating numerous bodily functions. It serves as a critical component of cells, tissues, and organs, enabling them to function optimally. Some key roles of water in the body include:

1. **Temperature regulation:** Water helps regulate body temperature through processes such as sweating and evaporative cooling.
2. **Nutrient absorption and waste removal:** Water facilitates the digestion, absorption, and transportation of nutrients throughout the body. It also aids in the

elimination of waste products through urine and perspiration.

3. **Lubrication and cushioning:** Water acts as a lubricant for joints, allowing smooth movement, and cushions organs and tissues, protecting them from impact and friction.
4. **Electrolyte balance:** Water helps maintain the balance of electrolytes, such as sodium, potassium, and magnesium, which are essential for proper muscle and nerve function.
5. **Transportation of oxygen and nutrients:** Water is a key component of blood, assisting in the transportation of oxygen, hormones, and nutrients to various cells and tissues.

B. Signs and Risks of Dehydration:
Dehydration occurs when the body loses more fluids than it takes in, resulting in an imbalance that can have negative effects on health. Common signs of dehydration include:

1. **Thirst:** Feeling thirsty is one of the initial indicators that your body needs more fluids.
2. **Dry mouth and lips:** A dry mouth and lips can be a sign of inadequate hydration.
3. **Dark-colored urine:** Urine that is darker in color, or a reduced frequency of urination, may indicate dehydration.
4. **Fatigue and weakness:** Dehydration can lead to feelings of tiredness, lack of energy, and reduced physical performance.

5. **Dizziness and lightheadedness:** Insufficient hydration can cause dizziness or lightheadedness, affecting balance and coordination.

6. **Headaches and difficulty concentrating:** Dehydration can contribute to headaches, difficulty concentrating, and impaired cognitive function.

Chronic dehydration can have more severe consequences and may increase the risk of urinary tract infections, kidney stones, constipation, and heat-related illnesses.

C. Tips for Staying Hydrated:

To maintain proper hydration throughout the day, consider the following tips:

1. **Drink an adequate amount of water:** Aim to consume the recommended daily intake of water, which is around 8 cups (64 ounces) for most individuals. This amount can vary based on factors such as age, activity level, and climate.

2. **Listen to your body:** Pay attention to your body's signals of thirst and drink water whenever you feel thirsty.

3. **Carry a reusable water bottle:** Having a water bottle with you serves as a reminder to drink water regularly and makes it easily accessible.

4. **Set reminders:** If you tend to forget to drink water, set reminders on your phone or use hydration-tracking apps to prompt you to hydrate throughout the day.

5. **Include hydrating foods:** Many fruits and vegetables have high water content, such as watermelon, cucumbers, strawberries, and spinach. Including these in your diet can contribute to your overall hydration.
6. **Limit alcohol and caffeinated beverages:** Alcoholic and caffeinated beverages can have a diuretic effect, increasing fluid loss. Consume them in moderation and balance them with an adequate intake of water.

D. Benefits of Proper Hydration: Maintaining proper hydration offers numerous benefits for overall health and well-being. Some of these benefits include:

1. **Improved physical performance:** Adequate hydration is essential for optimal physical performance. It helps regulate body temperature, lubricate joints, and transport nutrients and oxygen to muscles, allowing for better endurance, strength, and overall athletic performance.
2. **Enhanced cognitive function:** Staying hydrated supports optimal brain function. Dehydration can impair cognitive abilities, including concentration, alertness, and short-term memory. By maintaining proper hydration, you can

promote mental clarity and focus.

3. **Healthy skin:** Hydration plays a crucial role in maintaining healthy skin. Sufficient water intake helps keep the skin moisturized, improves elasticity, and promotes a radiant complexion. It can also help reduce the appearance of wrinkles and fine lines.

4. **Digestive health:** Water is essential for proper digestion and prevents common digestive issues such as constipation. Sufficient hydration softens stool, making it easier to pass, and supports the overall functioning of the digestive system.

5. **Detoxification:** Proper hydration aids in the elimination of toxins from the body through urine and sweat. It helps flush out waste products and supports the optimal functioning of the kidneys and liver, which are responsible for detoxification processes.

6. **Regulation of appetite:** Sometimes, thirst can be mistaken for hunger. By staying adequately hydrated, you can help differentiate between thirst and hunger cues, which may assist in maintaining healthy body weight and managing food intake.

7. **Joint and muscle health:** Water acts as a

lubricant for joints and helps prevent friction and discomfort. It also supports the delivery of nutrients to muscles and helps prevent muscle cramps and fatigue during physical activity. Hydration is essential for maintaining optimal health and well-being. By understanding the role of water in the body, recognizing signs of dehydration, and implementing strategies to stay hydrated, we can reap the benefits of proper hydration. From improved physical performance and cognitive function to healthy skin and digestive health, water plays a fundamental role in supporting various bodily functions. Prioritizing hydration as part of your daily routine will contribute to your overall vitality and promote a healthier, more vibrant life.

Chapter 4: The Power of Antioxidants: Protecting Against Free Radicals and Chronic Diseases

In our modern world, our bodies are constantly exposed to various environmental factors that can generate harmful molecules called free radicals. Free radicals can cause damage to cells and contribute to the development of chronic diseases. However, our bodies have a natural defense system against these harmful molecules in the form of antioxidants.

A. Understanding Free Radicals:

Free radicals are unstable molecules that have an unpaired electron in their outer shell. This makes them highly reactive and prone to stealing electrons from other molecules in the body, causing oxidative damage. Free radicals can be generated through various sources such as pollution, cigarette smoke, UV radiation, and even normal metabolic processes in the body.

B. The Role of Antioxidants:

Antioxidants are molecules that can neutralize free radicals by donating an electron without becoming unstable themselves. They act as scavengers, preventing free radicals from causing further damage to cells and tissues. Antioxidants can be produced naturally in the body, but they can also be obtained through diet by consuming antioxidant-rich foods.

C. Benefits of Antioxidants:

1. Protection against oxidative stress:

Oxidative stress occurs when there is an imbalance between the production of free radicals and the body's ability to neutralize them with antioxidants. Prolonged oxidative stress can contribute to chronic diseases such as cardiovascular disease, cancer, neurodegenerative disorders, and accelerated aging. Antioxidants play a crucial role in reducing oxidative stress and protecting against these diseases.

2. Boosting the immune system:

Antioxidants support a healthy immune system by protecting immune cells from oxidative damage. This helps to strengthen the immune response and enhance the body's ability to fight off infections and diseases.

3. Anti-inflammatory properties: Chronic inflammation is linked to the development of various diseases, including heart disease, diabetes, and certain cancers. Antioxidants have anti-inflammatory properties that help reduce inflammation and its associated risks, promoting overall health and well-being.

4. Skin Health and Aging: Free radicals can damage collagen and elastin fibers in the skin, leading to wrinkles, sagging, and other signs of aging. Antioxidants help protect against this damage, promoting healthier, more youthful-looking skin.

D. Food Sources of Antioxidants: A wide range of foods contains antioxidants, and including them in your diet can provide substantial health benefits. Some antioxidant-rich foods include:

1. **Berries:** Blueberries, strawberries, raspberries, and blackberries are packed with antioxidants like anthocyanins and vitamin C.
2. **Dark leafy greens:** Spinach, kale, and Swiss chard are excellent sources of antioxidants such as vitamin E, vitamin C, and beta-carotene.
3. **Nuts and seeds:** Almonds, walnuts, flaxseeds, and chia seeds are rich in antioxidants, healthy fats, and other beneficial nutrients.
4. **Colorful fruits and vegetables:** Brightly colored

fruits and vegetables like oranges, tomatoes, carrots, and peppers contain a variety of antioxidants.

5. **Green tea:** Green tea contains catechins, a type of antioxidant known for its health-promoting properties.
6. **Dark chocolate:** Dark chocolate with a high percentage of cocoa solids is a delicious source of antioxidants, particularly flavonoids.

E. Incorporating Antioxidants into Your Diet:

To maximize the benefits of antioxidants, aim to incorporate a variety of antioxidant-rich foods into your daily diet. Here are some tips:

1. **Eat a colorful plate:** Include a diverse range of fruits and vegetables of varying colors in your meals. Different colors indicate the presence of different antioxidants, so by incorporating a rainbow of produce, you can ensure a broad spectrum of antioxidants in your diet.
2. **Opt for whole, unprocessed foods:** Whole grains, legumes, nuts, and seeds are not only rich in antioxidants but also provide additional nutritional benefits. Choose these foods over processed and refined options.
3. **Prioritize organic and locally sourced produce:** Organic fruits and vegetables tend to have higher antioxidant levels,

as they are grown without the use of synthetic pesticides and fertilizers. Locally sourced produce is also fresher and retains more antioxidants compared to those that have traveled long distances.

4. **Prepare antioxidant-rich meals:** Experiment with recipes that incorporate antioxidant-rich ingredients. For example, create colorful salads with a variety of vegetables and fruits, make antioxidant-packed smoothies, or include antioxidant-rich spices like turmeric, cinnamon, and ginger in your cooking.

5. **Consider supplementation:** In some cases, dietary supplements may be recommended to ensure adequate intake of antioxidants. However, it's important to consult with a healthcare professional before starting any supplementation regimen.

F. Lifestyle Factors for Maximizing Antioxidant Benefits:

In addition to a diet rich in antioxidants, certain lifestyle factors can maximize the benefits of antioxidants:

1. **Regular exercise:** Engaging in regular physical activity can increase the production of antioxidants in the body and enhance their effectiveness. Aim for a combination of cardiovascular exercise and

strength training for optimal results.

2. **Manage stress levels:** Chronic stress can contribute to increased free radical production. Practice stress management techniques such as meditation, yoga, deep breathing exercises, and engaging in hobbies or activities you enjoy.

3. **Avoid smoking and limit alcohol consumption:** Smoking and excessive alcohol consumption increase the production of free radicals in the body. Quit smoking and consume alcohol in moderation, if at all, to minimize oxidative damage.

4. **Protect against sun exposure:** Ultraviolet (UV) radiation from the sun can generate free radicals in the skin. Protect your skin by wearing sunscreen, seeking shade during peak sun hours, and wearing protective clothing, hats, and sunglasses.

Incorporating antioxidants into your diet and lifestyle can significantly contribute to protecting against free radicals and reducing the risk of chronic diseases. By understanding the role of antioxidants, consuming antioxidant-rich foods, and adopting healthy lifestyle habits, you can unlock the power of antioxidants for vibrant living. Prioritize a colorful and varied diet, engage in regular physical activity, manage stress, and protect yourself from environmental factors that contribute to oxidative stress. Embrace the power of antioxidants and take proactive steps towards maintaining optimal health and well-being.

Chapter 5: Superfoods: Nutrient-Rich Foods for Optimal Health

Superfoods are a category of nutrient-dense foods that are exceptionally rich in vitamins, minerals, antioxidants, and other beneficial compounds. These foods have gained popularity for their potential to enhance overall health, boost immune function, support weight management, and reduce the risk of chronic diseases.

The Characteristics of Superfoods: Superfoods are characterized by their exceptional nutrient density, meaning they provide a high concentration of essential vitamins, minerals, and other health-promoting compounds while being relatively low in calories. These foods are typically rich in antioxidants, fiber, healthy fats, and phytochemicals, which are compounds found in plants that offer various health benefits.

A. Key Superfoods and Their Benefits:

1. Blueberries:
Blueberries are packed with antioxidants, particularly anthocyanins, which give them their vibrant color. These antioxidants help protect against oxidative damage, support brain health, reduce

inflammation, and enhance heart health. Blueberries are also a good source of fiber, vitamin C, and vitamin K.

2. Kale:

Kale is a nutrient powerhouse, rich in vitamins A, C, and K, as well as minerals like calcium, potassium, and magnesium. It is also a great source of antioxidants, including lutein and zeaxanthin, which promote eye health. Kale offers anti-inflammatory benefits, supports cardiovascular health, and provides a good amount of fiber.

3. Salmon:

Salmon is an excellent source of omega-3 fatty acids, particularly EPA and DHA, which are essential for brain health and reducing inflammation. It is also rich in high-quality protein, vitamin D, and B vitamins. Consuming salmon regularly can support heart health, improve cognitive function, and promote healthy skin.

4. Quinoa:

Quinoa is a gluten-free grain that is highly nutritious and packed with protein, fiber, and various minerals such as magnesium, iron, and zinc. It is also a good source of antioxidants and contains all nine essential amino acids, making it a complete protein. Quinoa supports healthy digestion, provides sustained energy, and contributes to satiety.

5. Chia Seeds:

Chia seeds are a nutritional powerhouse, loaded with fiber, omega-3 fatty acids, protein, and antioxidants. They also provide calcium, magnesium, and phosphorus. Chia seeds support digestive health, promote heart health, stabilize blood sugar levels, and aid in weight management.

B. Incorporating Superfoods into Your Diet:

To reap the benefits of superfoods, consider the following tips for incorporating them into your diet:

- **Variety is key:** Aim to include a diverse range of superfoods in your meals to maximize nutritional benefits. Experiment with different fruits, vegetables, grains, and proteins to discover new favorites.
- **Smoothies and bowls:** Blend superfoods like berries, kale, and chia seeds into smoothies or create nutrient-rich bowls with a base of quinoa or whole grains topped with colorful fruits and vegetables.
- **Salads and stir-fries:** Add superfoods such as spinach, kale, avocado, and nuts to salads and stir-fries for an extra nutritional boost.
- **Snack smart:** Replace processed snacks with superfood options like mixed nuts, trail mix, or fresh fruit to satisfy cravings while nourishing your body.
- **Superfood swaps:** Substitute ingredients in recipes with superfood alternatives. For example, use quinoa instead of rice or incorporate chia seeds into baking recipes.
- **Plan:** Prepare meals and snacks in advance, incorporating superfoods, so

you have convenient and healthy options readily available. This can include prepping salads with nutrient-rich ingredients, making overnight chia seed pudding, or roasting a batch of kale chips for on-the-go snacking.

- **Explore recipes:** Look for recipes that specifically highlight superfoods as main ingredients or incorporate them creatively. There are countless resources available, including cookbooks, websites, and food blogs dedicated to showcasing delicious ways to enjoy superfoods.

- **Seasonal eating:** Embrace seasonal produce as many fresh fruits and vegetables are considered superfoods. Not only does this support local agriculture, but it also ensures that you're consuming produce at its peak nutritional value.

- **Superfood combinations:** Combine different superfoods to create a power-packed meal or snack. For instance, top a bowl of Greek yogurt with blueberries, chia seeds, and a sprinkle of almonds for a balanced and nutrient-rich breakfast.

- **Moderation and balance:** While superfoods offer numerous health benefits, it's important to remember that a balanced diet is key. Incorporate superfoods alongside a variety of other nutrient-dense foods to ensure you're getting a wide range of essential nutrients.

Superfoods provide a fantastic opportunity to enhance your diet with nutrient-rich ingredients that offer a plethora of health benefits. By incorporating superfoods like blueberries, kale, salmon, quinoa, and chia seeds into your meals and snacks, you can boost your nutrient intake, support overall health, and promote vibrant living. Experiment with different superfoods, try new recipes and enjoy the incredible flavors and benefits these foods have to offer. Remember to maintain a balanced approach to your diet and combine superfoods with a variety of other wholesome ingredients for optimal nutrition and well-being.

C. Creating a Balanced Plate: The Basics of Meal Planning

Meal planning is a valuable tool for promoting healthy eating habits, achieving nutritional balance, and ensuring that your meals are nourishing and satisfying.

1. The Benefits of Meal Planning:

- **Nutritional balance:** Meal planning allows you to create balanced meals that include a variety of food groups, ensuring you get a range of essential nutrients. This promotes optimal health and supports your body's needs.
- **Cost-effective:** Meal planning can help you make smart choices when grocery shopping, prevent food waste, and minimize impulsive

purchases. This can lead to significant cost savings over time.

- **Healthier choices:** With a meal plan in place, you're less likely to rely on convenience foods or unhealthy takeout options. By intentionally selecting nutritious ingredients, you can make healthier choices and avoid the temptation of less nutritious alternatives.

2. The Components of a Balanced Plate:

A balanced plate consists of the following components:

- **Protein:** Choose lean sources of protein such as poultry, fish, legumes, tofu, or tempeh. Protein is essential for building and repairing tissues, supporting immune function, and providing a feeling of fullness.
- **Whole grains:** Opt for whole grains like brown rice, quinoa, whole wheat bread, or oats. Whole grains provide fiber, vitamins, minerals, and sustained energy.
- **Vegetables:** Include a variety of colorful vegetables to maximize nutrient intake. Aim to fill half of your plate with non-starchy vegetables such as leafy greens, broccoli, bell peppers, carrots, or zucchini.
- **Fruits:** Incorporate fresh or frozen fruits to add natural sweetness, fiber, and vitamins to your meals. Enjoy them as a

side dish, snack, or as part of a balanced dessert.

- **Healthy fats:** Include sources of healthy fats like avocados, nuts, seeds, olive oil, or fatty fish. These fats provide essential fatty acids, support brain health, and help absorb fat-soluble vitamins.

3. Meal Planning Strategies:

- **Plan your meals:** Set aside time each week to plan your meals and create a shopping list accordingly. Consider your schedule, dietary preferences, and any specific nutritional goals or dietary restrictions.

- **Batch cooking:** Prepare larger quantities of food and portion them out for multiple meals. This saves time during the week and ensures you have healthy options readily available.

- **Use a variety of cooking methods:** Experiment with different cooking methods such as grilling, baking, sautéing, or steaming to add variety and enhance flavors to your meals.

- **Embrace leftovers:** Plan for leftovers by intentionally cooking extra servings. Leftovers can be used for lunches or repurposed into new meals, reducing food waste and saving time.

- **Have a go-to list of recipes:** Compile a collection of favorite recipes that are balanced, nutritious, and easy to prepare. Having a list of go-to recipes simplifies meal planning and ensures variety in your meals.

4. Customizing Your Meal Plan:

- **Consider your individual needs:** Take into account your specific dietary requirements, preferences, and any health conditions when creating your meal plan. Customize it to fit your unique needs.

- **Portion control:** Pay attention to portion sizes to avoid overeating. Use visual cues, such as using your hand as a guide for appropriate portion sizes. For example, a serving of protein should be about the size of your palm, while a serving of grains or starchy vegetables can fit in your cupped hand.

- **Listen to your body:** Tune in to your hunger and fullness cues when planning and consuming meals. This helps you maintain a healthy relationship with food and eat according to your body's needs.

- **Seek variety:** Incorporate a diverse range of foods from different food groups to ensure you're getting a wide array of nutrients. Experiment with new ingredients, flavors, and cooking techniques to keep your meals exciting and enjoyable.

- **Plan for snacks:** Don't forget to include nutritious snacks in your meal plan to keep your energy levels stable

throughout the day. Choose
snacks that combine protein,
fiber, and healthy fats to
provide sustained energy and
satiety.

- **Be flexible:** While meal
  planning provides structure, it's
  important to remain flexible
  and adaptable. Allow room for
  spontaneity, special occasions,
  and dining out while making
  mindful choices that align with
  your overall health goals.

Meal planning is a valuable tool for
creating balanced, nutritious meals
and supporting your overall health and
well-being. By incorporating protein,
whole grains, vegetables, fruits, and
healthy fats into your meals, you can
ensure a well-rounded plate that
provides a variety of essential
nutrients. Customize your meal plan to
fit your individual needs, listen to your
body's cues, and seek variety in your
food choices. With proper planning
and a balanced plate, you can enjoy
the benefits of nutritious meals, save
time and money, and make positive
strides toward vibrant living.

Chapter 6. Cooking and Food Preparation Techniques for Nutrient Retention

A. Cooking and food preparation

The way we cook and prepare our
food can have a significant impact on
the nutritional content and overall

health benefits of the meals we consume. By understanding these techniques, you can optimize the nutritional value of your meals and support your journey towards healthy eating and vibrant living.

1. Steaming:
Steaming is a gentle cooking method that involves using steam to cook food. This technique helps retain the nutrients in vegetables, preserving their vibrant colors and crisp texture. Steaming is especially effective for heat-sensitive nutrients like vitamins C and B vitamins. To steam food, place it in a steamer basket or a colander over boiling water and cover it with a lid. Steam until the food is tender yet still retains its nutritional value.

2. Stir-Frying:
Stir-frying involves quickly cooking food in a small amount of oil over high heat. This technique is popular in Asian cuisine and allows for the retention of nutrients due to the short cooking time. Stir-frying uses a variety of colorful vegetables and can be combined with lean protein sources for a well-balanced meal. To stir-fry, heat a small amount of oil in a wok or skillet, add your ingredients, and cook them quickly while continuously stirring.

3. Grilling:
Grilling is a cooking method that adds a smoky flavor to food while retaining its nutritional value. It is particularly suitable for lean meats, fish, and vegetables. When grilling, marinate the ingredients beforehand to add flavor and protect them from charring. Opt for lower temperatures and avoid

excessive charring, as it can produce potentially harmful compounds. Additionally, consider using a marinade with acidic ingredients like lemon juice or vinegar, as they can help reduce the formation of harmful compounds during grilling.

4. Roasting:

Roasting involves cooking food in the oven at a high temperature. This technique brings out the natural flavors and textures of ingredients while preserving their nutrients. Roasting is great for root vegetables, poultry, fish, and certain fruits. To roast food, toss it in a small amount of oil and seasonings, spread it out on a baking sheet, and cook it in the oven until it is golden and tender.

5. Blending and Pureeing:

Blending and pureeing are methods commonly used for making smoothies, soups, and sauces. These techniques involve combining ingredients in a blender or food processor until they reach a smooth consistency. Blending and pureeing help break down the cell walls of fruits and vegetables, making their nutrients more readily available for absorption. By using whole fruit or vegetable, including the skin and fiber-rich parts, you maximize the nutritional content.

6. Raw Preparation:

Consuming fruits and vegetables in their raw state is an excellent way to preserve their natural nutrients. Raw foods provide enzymes, vitamins, and antioxidants that may be diminished through cooking. Incorporate raw ingredients into salads, wraps, or as crunchy snacks. However, keep in mind that some vegetables, such as tomatoes and carrots, have enhanced nutrient availability when cooked. A combination of raw and cooked foods can provide a balance of nutrients and flavors.

7. Proper Storage and Minimal Processing:

Proper storage and minimal processing techniques are crucial for preserving the nutritional value of ingredients. Store fruits and vegetables in the refrigerator to slow down nutrient loss. Minimize exposure to air, light, and heat, as they can degrade vitamins and antioxidants. Additionally, avoid overprocessing foods, as excessive chopping, peeling, and extended cooking can lead to nutrient loss.

The way we cook and prepare our food plays a significant role in the retention of nutrients and the overall nutritional value of our meals. By utilizing cooking and food preparation techniques such as steaming, stir-frying, grilling, roasting, blending, and raw preparation, we can maximize nutrient retention in our ingredients. These techniques help preserve the vibrant colors, flavors, and textures of the food while ensuring that essential vitamins, minerals, and antioxidants remain intact.

It is also important to practice proper storage methods and minimize processing to maintain the nutritional integrity of ingredients. By storing fruits and vegetables correctly and avoiding excessive chopping, peeling, and extended cooking, we can minimize nutrient loss and preserve the natural goodness of our food.

By incorporating these cooking and food preparation techniques into our daily lives, we can create meals that are not only delicious but also packed with essential nutrients. Experiment with different methods, explore new flavors and textures and embrace the variety of nutrient-rich ingredients available to us. With mindful cooking and preparation, we can unlock the full potential of our food and embark on a journey towards healthy eating and vibrant living.

Remember, nutrition is a multifaceted aspect of overall well-being, and combining these cooking techniques with a balanced and varied diet will provide the foundation for optimal health and vitality.

B. Eating on a Budget: Making Nutritious Choices Affordably

Eating a nutritious diet doesn't have to break the bank. With strategic planning, smart shopping, and budget-friendly meal ideas, it is possible to make healthy and nutritious choices while sticking to a budget.

1. Prioritize Whole Foods:

When budgeting for nutritious eating, prioritize whole foods over processed and packaged options. Whole foods such as fruits, vegetables, whole grains, legumes, and lean proteins provide a wealth of essential nutrients at a lower cost. These foods are often less expensive, especially when purchased in bulk or season, and offer more value for your money.

2. Plan Meals and Create a Shopping List:

Meal planning is a powerful tool for cost-effective and nutritious eating. Plan your meals, considering ingredients that can be used in multiple dishes and making use of leftovers. By creating a shopping list based on your meal plan, you can avoid impulse purchases and ensure you only buy what you need, minimizing food waste and overspending.

3. Shop Smart:

Consider these strategies when shopping to stretch your budget further:

- **Compare prices:** Compare prices at different grocery stores and consider buying generic or store-brand items, as they are often more affordable without compromising quality.
- **Buy in bulk:** Purchase non-perishable items, such as grains, beans, nuts, and seeds, in bulk. This can be more cost-effective and allows you to portion them as needed.
- **Utilize frozen and canned options:** Frozen fruits and vegetables and canned beans, tuna, and tomatoes are often less expensive than their fresh counterparts and can be just as nutritious. They also have a longer shelf life, reducing waste.
- **Check for sales and discounts:** Keep an eye out for sales, promotions, and discounts on nutritious foods.

Plan your meals around these deals to save money.

- **Stick to the perimeter:** The perimeter of the grocery store typically houses fresh produce, meat, and dairy products. Focus on these areas as they tend to offer healthier and more affordable options compared to the processed and packaged foods found in the middle aisles.

4. Cook and Prepare Meals at Home:

Cooking and preparing meals at home is not only more cost-effective but also allows you to have control over the ingredients you use. Explore simple and budget-friendly recipes that utilize affordable staples like rice, beans, lentils, and seasonal produce. Cooking in batches and utilizing leftovers for subsequent meals can further stretch your budget and save time.

5. Embrace Plant-Based Proteins:

Plant-based proteins such as beans, lentils, tofu, and tempeh are often more affordable than meat and poultry. Incorporate these protein sources into your meals to reduce costs while still meeting your nutritional needs. Experiment with flavorful recipes and spices to make plant-based proteins delicious and satisfying.

6. Minimize Food Waste:

Reducing food waste is not only environmentally friendly but also helps save money. Plan your meals based on the ingredients you already have on hand and utilize leftovers creatively. Use vegetable scraps for homemade stocks, repurpose cooked grains and vegetables into salads or stir-fries, and freeze excess produce for future use.

7. Grow Your Food:

Consider starting a small herb garden or growing your fruits and vegetables, even if you have limited space. Growing your food can be cost-effective, and rewarding, and provides access to fresh, nutritious produce right at your doorstep.

Eating well on a budget is entirely possible with careful planning, strategic shopping, and smart choices. Prioritize whole foods, plan your meals, shop smartly, cook at home, and embrace cost-effective options like plant-based proteins. By minimizing food waste and exploring creative ways to use ingredients, you can stretch your budget while still nourishing your body with nutritious meals.

Remember, eating on a budget doesn't mean sacrificing taste or quality. With a little creativity and resourcefulness, you can discover delicious and affordable recipes that incorporate wholesome ingredients. Take advantage of sales, discounts, and bulk purchases, and be mindful of the value that whole foods offer in terms of nutrition and cost.

Additionally, consider the long-term benefits of growing your food, even if it's just a small herb garden or a few potted plants. Not only does it save money, but it also provides a rewarding and sustainable way to access fresh produce.

By implementing these strategies and making conscious choices, you can maintain a nutritious and balanced diet while adhering to your budgetary constraints. Eating well doesn't have to be an expensive endeavor. With planning, creativity, and a focus on whole, affordable foods, you can make nutritious choices that support your health and financial well-being. Remember, the key is to find a balance that works for you and your budget. By making small changes and adopting these cost-effective practices, you can achieve a healthy and vibrant lifestyle without breaking the bank.

Chapter 7: Understanding Food Labels and Making Informed Choices

Food labels provide valuable information about the nutritional content and ingredients of packaged foods. Understanding how to read and interpret food labels is essential for making informed choices that align with your health goals.

A. Serving Size and Servings per Container:

The serving size is the recommended amount of the food product to consume, and the servings per container indicate how many servings are in the entire package. Pay attention to these values, as they determine the nutritional information provided on the label and help you gauge your intake accurately.

B. Ingredient List:
The ingredient list provides valuable insights into the composition of the food product. Ingredients are listed in descending order by weight, with the most abundant ingredient listed first. Be aware of any additives, preservatives, or artificial ingredients that may be present. Aim for products with a shorter ingredient list and prioritize whole, recognizable ingredients.

C. Allergens and Special Dietary Needs:
Food labels also indicate if the product contains common allergens such as gluten, soy, dairy, nuts, or shellfish. If you have specific dietary restrictions or allergies, carefully review the allergen information to ensure the product is safe for consumption.

D. Health Claims and Marketing Terminology:
Be cautious of health claims and marketing terminology on food labels. Some terms may be misleading or used as marketing strategies. Always refer to the actual nutritional information and ingredient list to make informed decisions about the product's suitability for your dietary needs.

E. Organic and Non-GMO Labels:
If you are interested in organic or non-genetically modified organism (GMO) foods, look for specific labels indicating organic certification or non-GMO verification. These labels ensure that the product has met certain standards and guidelines.

F. Comparing and Analyzing Food Labels:

To make informed choices, compare food labels of different products within the same category. Pay attention to the nutrient content, ingredient list, and serving sizes. This allows you to select products that align with your nutritional goals and preferences. Understanding food labels empowers you to make informed choices about the foods you consume. By analyzing serving sizes, nutrient content, ingredient lists, and allergen information, you can select products that support your dietary needs and health goals. Be mindful of marketing claims and focus on the actual nutritional information provided on the label.

Developing label-reading skills helps you navigate the grocery store with confidence, ensuring that the foods you purchase align with your values and contribute to your overall well-being. By making informed choices, you can cultivate a nutritious and balanced diet that promotes vibrant living.

G. Mindful Eating: Cultivating a Healthy Relationship with Food

In our fast-paced world, it's easy to fall into patterns of mindless eating and disconnectedness from our food. By adopting mindful eating principles, we can enhance our overall well-being, improve digestion, and develop a greater appreciation for the nourishment that food provides.

1. The Basics of Mindful Eating:

Mindful eating involves bringing full awareness to the eating experience, engaging all our senses, and being present at the moment. By paying attention to our body's hunger and fullness cues, we can better respond to its needs and make conscious choices about what, when, and how much to eat.

2. Honoring Hunger and Fullness:
Recognizing our body's hunger and fullness signals is crucial for mindful eating. Before eating, pause and assess your level of hunger. Eat when you are moderately hungry rather than ravenous, and stop eating when you are comfortably satisfied, but not overly full. Tune in to your body's cues and respect its natural signals of satiety.

3. Slowing Down and Savoring Each Bite:
Eating slowly allows us to fully experience the flavors, textures, and aromas of our food. Chew each bite thoroughly and savor the taste. This practice not only enhances our enjoyment of the meal but also supports proper digestion and satiety awareness.

4. Engaging the Senses:
Engage all your senses when eating. Notice the colors, textures, and smells of the food. Take time to appreciate the presentation and the effort that went into preparing the meal. By involving all your senses, you can enhance the pleasure and satisfaction derived from eating.

5. Mindful Food Choices:
When making food choices, practice mindfulness by considering the nutritional value and how different foods make you feel. Aim for a balance of macronutrients and include a variety of colorful fruits, vegetables,

whole grains, and lean proteins in your meals. Be aware of portion sizes and choose foods that nourish your body and support your well-being.

6. Emotional Eating:
Emotional eating often involves using food to cope with emotions rather than responding to true hunger. Mindful eating encourages us to develop an awareness of our emotions and find alternative ways to address them without relying on food. Engage in activities such as journaling, exercising, or seeking support from loved ones to manage emotional well-being.

7. Mindful Eating in Everyday Life:
Extend the practice of mindful eating beyond mealtimes. Bring awareness to your snacking habits and the consumption of beverages. Choose nutritious snacks mindfully, paying attention to portion sizes and how they contribute to your overall diet. Be present during moments of food-related socializing and practice mindful eating during these occasions as well.

8. Gratitude and Appreciation:
Express gratitude for the food you have and the nourishment it provides. Cultivate a sense of appreciation for the farmers, producers, and everyone involved in bringing food to your table. Recognize the interconnectedness of food and its impact on your well-being, fostering a deeper sense of gratitude and connection.

Mindful eating is a transformative practice that allows us to establish a healthier relationship with food. By slowing down, paying attention to our

body's cues, and engaging our
senses, we can savor the joy and
nourishment that each meal brings.
Mindful eating not only enhances our
physical health but also promotes
emotional well-being, self-awareness,
and gratitude.
Incorporate mindful eating principles
into your daily life, one bite at a time.
Practice awareness, gratitude, and
conscious decision-making when it
comes to food choices. Be patient with
yourself as you develop this new
approach to eating, as it may take
time to break old habits and fully
embrace mindful eating.
Remember, mindful eating is not
about perfection or restriction. It's
about creating a positive and balanced
relationship with food that supports
your overall well-being. Be
compassionate towards yourself and
allow for flexibility in your choices,
finding a middle ground between
nourishing your body and enjoying the
foods you love.
As you continue on your mindful
eating journey, you may notice
improvements in digestion, increased
satisfaction from meals, and a
heightened sense of self-awareness
around your eating habits. Embrace
these positive changes and celebrate
the progress you make along the way.
Incorporating mindfulness into your
eating habits can extend to other
areas of your life as well. The practice
of being present, appreciating the little
things, and savoring each moment
can enhance your overall mindfulness
and bring a sense of calm and
balance to your daily routines.

By cultivating a healthy relationship with food through mindful eating, you are not only nourishing your body but also fostering a deeper connection with yourself and the world around you. Embrace the transformative power of mindful eating and enjoy the journey towards vibrant and mindful living.

Remember, each meal is an opportunity to nourish your body and feed your soul. Approach it with gratitude, awareness, and a sense of joy, knowing that you are taking steps towards a healthier and more fulfilling lifestyle through the practice of mindful eating.

Conclusion:

In this comprehensive guide to healthy eating and vibrant living, we have explored the power of nutrition and its profound impact on our health and well-being. Each chapter has delved into various aspects of nutrition, providing valuable information, insights, and practical tips to help readers make informed choices and embrace a healthier lifestyle.

From understanding macronutrients and micronutrients to exploring the importance of fiber, hydration, antioxidants, and superfoods, we have uncovered the key components of a balanced and nutritious diet. We have learned about the importance of mindful eating, the gut-brain connection, and the role of nutrition in different life stages and performance.

We have also discussed practical considerations such as meal planning, food preparation techniques, eating on a budget, and decoding food labels. Additionally, we have debunked myths surrounding diets and fad diets, empowering readers to make choices based on evidence-based nutrition principles.

Throughout this guide, we have emphasized the significance of sustainability and individualization in achieving long-term success. Rather than focusing on quick fixes or rigid rules, we have encouraged readers to adopt a holistic approach to nutrition, taking into account their unique needs, preferences, and goals.

Building healthy habits and sustaining long-term dietary changes require dedication, patience, and a supportive environment. It is a journey of self-discovery, self-care, and self-improvement. By embracing a balanced and mindful approach to eating, incorporating regular physical activity, and fostering a positive relationship with food, readers can unlock the power of nutrition and experience vibrant living.

Remember, healthy eating is not about deprivation or perfection. It is about nourishing our bodies, fueling our lives, and finding joy in the process. As you embark on your journey towards better nutrition and vibrant living, may this guide serve as a valuable resource and companion, empowering you to make choices that enhance your health, well-being, and overall quality of life. Here's to a

healthier, happier, and more vibrant
you!